MY PARENT HAS AN

AUTISM
SPECTRUM
DISORDER

of related interest

Something Different About Dad
How to Live With Your Asperger's Parent
Kirsti Evans and John Swogger
ISBN 978 1 84905 114 9

A Book About What Autism Can Be Like
Sue Adams
ISBN 978 1 84310 940 2

MY PARENT HAS AN
AUTISM
SPECTRUM
DISORDER

A Workbook for Children & Teens

Barbara R. Lester

Jessica Kingsley Publishers
London and Philadelphia

First published in 2011
by Jessica Kingsley Publishers
116 Pentonville Road
London N1 9JB, UK
and
400 Market Street, Suite 400
Philadelphia, PA 19106, USA
www.jkp.com

Library of Congress Cataloging in Publication Data
A CIP catalog record for this book is available from the Library of Congress

British Library Cataloguing in Publication Data
A CIP catalogue record for this book is available from the British Library

ISBN 978 1 84905 835 3

Printed and bound in Great Britain by
MPG Books Group

This book is dedicated to my mother
Ruth Luvenia Frye Lester
who always believed in me

Contents

Acknowledgments

I thank my father for teaching me so many things. Now, at the age of 89, he is teaching me how to share the end of someone's life. I thank my mother for always believing in me. I like to think she is watching over her family still. I thank my sister Patricia Kathryn Brussard for sharing the grand adventure of our family life.

Heartfelt thanks go to my amazing husband, Kerry Taylor, who always stands by me and steadies the family ship no matter how zany my plans or how windy the storm. He has had to take over many things at home while I have spent my weekends plugging away at this book. I have gratitude for my three wonderful children, Dusty Swede, Travis Swede, and Sean Taylor, who have helped me become who I am. I hope I have helped you become who you are too.

I thank the hundreds of clients and their families that I have worked with over the years, especially those who are affected by autism spectrum disorders. I have learned so much while sharing your life journeys with you. I cannot thank you personally since I must keep your stories private.

I thank my wonderful colleagues and the staff of Primary Children's Center for Counseling in Salt Lake City, Utah. I greatly appreciate your friendship and support. I learn new things from you every day.

I owe a hug and a rosary to all of my friends at the Cathedral of the Madeleine in Salt Lake City where my soul gets restored every week. I can't imagine my life without all of you and without all the inspiring music. Thanks be to God.

My thanks as well to Jessica Kingsley and all of her staff, including Cerys Owen, Helen Ibbotson, Alexandra Higson, and Rachel Menzies. I hope that by publishing this book we are able to provide additional support to children, teens, and families affected by autism spectrum disorders.

I am writing this book to my younger self—I could have used the advice back when I was growing up! So here's to the next generation—please make a wonderful world for yourselves and pay it forwards. I can't wait to see the contributions you will make.

Chapter 1

About You

You are reading this book because you have a parent who has an autism spectrum disorder. From now on to make things easier we will call an autism spectrum disorder an "ASD" for short. You may have recently found out about the ASD, or you may have known for a long time. You probably have questions you would like answered. You may want to understand your parent better. You and your parent may have problems getting along at times that you both would like to solve. You may be wondering if there are other children or teens who face any of the same issues in their families that you do in yours. You may be experiencing some special stresses from being in a family affected by an ASD. You may know that your ASD parent has special strengths and talents but wonder if anyone appreciates those strengths or if they only notice the weaknesses.

This first chapter will show how your questions about ASDs will be answered in the rest of the book. Most of the chapters begin with a few paragraphs for you to read and then end with a worksheet that you can complete with your family. By doing the worksheets together you can all learn more about each other and develop skills for solving any ASD-related problems. In Chapter 2, you will read about how I grew up with an ASD parent and how I learned enough about ASDs to be able to write this book.

Chapter 3 answers questions on what ASDs are all about, such as "What exactly is an ASD?", "What causes an ASD?", and "How do people find out that they have an ASD?"

Chapter 4 answers questions about social activities and parties, such as "Why doesn't my parent like to go to social events with me?", "What is it like for someone with an ASD to be at a party and have so many other people around?", and "How can my parent and I find social activities we both enjoy?"

Chapter 5 answers questions about conversations and figures of speech, such as "Why does my parent take things so literally?", "Why does my parent misunderstand some figures of speech?", and "What can I do to get a turn to talk?"

Chapter 6 answers questions about special interests, such as "Why is my parent so intense about his or her interests?", "Why isn't my parent more interested in the things that are important to me?", and "What are some of the good things about my parent's special interests?"

Chapter 7 answers questions about empathy and understanding others, such as "Why doesn't my parent understand my feelings very well?", "Why doesn't my parent seem to care what other people think?", and "What can I do when I want my parent to understand my point of view better?"

Chapter 8 answers questions about body language, such as "Why doesn't my parent show many facial expressions?", "Why does my parent misunderstand what I mean at times?", and "What can someone do to learn more about body language?"

Chapter 9 answers questions about emotions, such as "Why does my parent get worried so often?", "Why does my parent sometimes have strong feelings about little problems?", and "How can someone get help if they have problems with their emotions?"

Chapter 10 answers questions about learning, organizing, and appearance, such as "Why does my parent tell me every detail of something that has happened, instead of just the main point?", "Sometimes my family is disorganized—how can we get things done on time?", and "What can I do if I am worried about how my parent will dress at a special event?"

Chapter 11 answers questions about humor and imagination, such as "What can I do when my parent doesn't get my jokes?", "Why doesn't my parent understand my friends when they are being sarcastic?", and "How could my parent learn more about humor?"

Chapter 12 answers questions about rules and routines, such as "Why does my parent have to do things in a certain order?", "Why does my parent act like a police officer at home and try to get us to follow the rules?", and "What can we do as a family when my parent's routines aren't working for the rest of us?"

Chapter 13 answers questions about playing games and sports, such as "Why does my parent get so upset over losing a game?", "Why are some people with ASDs uncoordinated?", and "What kind of games could my parent and I enjoy playing together?"

Chapter 14 answers questions about sensory issues, such as "Why does my parent get so easily irritated by sounds?", "Why does my parent only like to wear clothes made of certain material?", and "What can I do to help my parent when sensory problems are bothering him or her?"

Chapter 15 answers questions about what would be appropriate to tell friends, such as "Why do we tell some people but not others about the ASD?", "Why do some people keep the ASD diagnosis private?", and "What should I do if my friends ask questions about my parent being different?"

The last chapter, Chapter 16, answers questions about special strengths and contributions of people with ASDs, such as "What are the strengths of people with ASDs?", "Who are some famous people with ASDs?", and "What are the positive things about my parent having an ASD?"

There are things your family can do to understand you and the questions you might have about ASDs. Fill out the worksheet below and show it to your family, so they can learn about you and what you think is important.

These are the things I like best at school: _____

_____

These are the things I like least at school: _____

_____

These are my closest friends: _____

_____

These are my favorite ways to spend free time: _____

_____

_____

Here are some of the best things about me: _____

_____

_____

_____

Here are some of the problems I have at times: _____

_____

_____

_____

My favorite vacation was: _____

I would like to accomplish these goals in my future: _____

_____

_____

_____

These are some of the questions I have about ASDs: _____

_____

_____

_____

_____

Chapter 2

About the Author

In this chapter, I want you to get to know me, the author, so you can understand how I came to write this book. When I was growing up, there were things about my father that made him different than the other fathers I knew. The main thing I noticed was that he seemed to like his special interests better than people. The special interest that was most important to him was chess and he liked to teach me about the game and bring me to chess club meetings. Another of his special interests was food, and he liked finding special cook books and pots and pans for my mother so she could make his favorite foods. He also had a special interest in literature and classical music, and he liked to teach my sister about books and poetry and bring her to the opera. However, he did not seem to enjoy spending time with us doing our other activities. He did not socialize with my mother's friends from work when they came over to the house. He did not go to my horse shows or to my sister's dance recitals. He liked the people from his chess club as chess partners but rarely had them come over to our house to do things with the family. He had a best friend whom he could talk to for hours on the phone, but they mostly talked about chess, not about their personal lives. He did not spend time getting to know my friends if they came over to play. My friends often felt nervous around him and worried that he did not like them, since he did not show interest in them or ask them questions about themselves.

My father liked following routines and doing things in just a certain way. We knew when he was going to take a shower that he would be in the bathroom for about an hour, because he wanted to follow all the steps of his showering routine. We only had one bathroom, so sometimes his routine would be a problem! He would get nervous about traveling anywhere, because he would be afraid that he would not have enough time to do his shower routine on vacation. He also wanted to eat certain foods together, and if you did not have mint jelly with lamb, or apple sauce with pork, or vinegar with spinach he would get mad about it. If we went to a restaurant that made their milk shakes with soft serve ice cream instead of "real" ice cream, he would get mad about that too and would not drink the milk shake.

There were many more differences I noticed over the years, and I will give those examples in the chapters to come. What I did not know when I was growing up was that these differences had a name. I also did not know there were other people in the world who had similar differences. It was not until some other people in my family tree were diagnosed with ASDs that I realized that my father had an ASD too. Have you heard how when people figure out something that surprises them they say that a lightbulb went on? When other people in our family tree were diagnosed with ASDs a really big lightbulb went on for me! Now I had a name to describe how my father was different. I could now learn about ASDs and figure out some things about our family.

Before I knew about the ASDs in my family tree, I went to college to study psychology. Psychology is the study of human behavior. When I went to college, scientists did not yet know that approximately 1 out of every 110 people has an ASD. Back then, in the late 1970s, scientists thought that only 1 out of every 3000 people had an ASD! Therefore, even though I studied psychology, I was not taught much about ASDs because they were thought to be quite rare. After that, I went to graduate school to study social work. Social workers help others handle and solve problems to improve the quality of their lives. After I finished graduate school, I began my job as a social worker, working mostly with children, teenagers, and their parents.

A number of years later, when I found out about the ASDs in my family tree, I started doing more counseling for other families who had ASDs in their family trees. I realized that I had learned a great deal about ASDs without knowing it from growing up with my father, and that I already knew how to understand people who had ASDs from that experience. I began to study and learn more about ASDs so I could help my own family and other families. I created and taught a class for parents who had children with ASDs. I counseled children and teens with ASDs and discovered that many of their parents also had ASDs. I taught social skills classes for children and teens with ASDs, and I counseled siblings about what it is like to be in a family affected by ASDs. I also set up a website about ASD issues (www.asdspecialist.com) and a YouTube channel that has videos to help families affected by ASDs (ASDspecialist).

You and I have something in common. We both have a parent with an ASD. I hope that you can use this book to understand your parent better and to solve any problems that you are having due to growing up in a family affected by an ASD.

Chapter 3

What is an Autism Spectrum Disorder?

You are reading a book about what it means to have a parent with an ASD. One thing you might be wondering is what exactly an ASD is. The word "autism" comes from the Greek word "autos." The word "autos" does not mean car in Greek! It means "he himself" and it describes someone who is not aware of others or acts withdrawn from others. A very important thing to understand is that ASDs are *neurological* differences. Neurological means that the differences we are talking about are hardwired into how the brain and nervous system work and so the person with an ASD cannot choose to behave differently. A person who does not have an ASD is called a "neurotypical," who from now on we will call an "NT" for short. An NT's brain works in a "typical" or usual way. The brain of someone with an ASD works in an unusual (or "atypical") way that can cause some problems for that person. The problem part is why these differences are called "disorders." Quite a few people, however, do not think of autism spectrum differences as disorders, disabilities, or problems. Instead, they believe these differences are just part of the normal range of human differences.

Some people with ASDs have very mild differences from NTs and do not need any special help, while others have very large differences and may not be able to talk or care for themselves. The word "spectrum" means that there is this wide range of differences.

A person does not choose to have an ASD and at this time ASDs cannot be cured with medication or therapy. However, some of the problems caused by ASDs can be solved with the right kind of help. For instance, many of the very young ASD children who cannot talk do learn to talk by getting speech therapy when they are in preschool. Also, many children and teens with ASDs attend groups to improve their social skills. ASDs are not illnesses that are contagious, like cold viruses. Instead, it is believed that for the most part people are born with ASD wiring. You can sometimes tell by looking at someone if they have another type of disability (such as if they are in a wheelchair or if they are blind) but you cannot tell by looking at someone if they have an ASD. Sometimes not being able to see the difference makes it harder to understand that basic question of what exactly an ASD is.

Another question you may have is "What causes an ASD?" Scientists do not fully know the answer to that question yet. We do know that genetics is one main cause of ASDs. That means that your parent's ASD has probably been inherited from others further back in the family tree. Your parent might have inherited eye color from his or her father or curly hair from a grandmother or a long and lanky build from a great grandfather. If you have a parent with an ASD, chances are there are other family members further back in your family tree who had ASDs, even though no one knew at that time. There are many scientists studying the question of what causes ASDs, and there are many people with ASDs in their family trees who are taking part in research studies to help the scientists answer this question.

A third question you may have is "How many people have ASDs?" In 2010 (when I am writing this book), scientists are saying that about 1 in every 110 children has an ASD. This means that if you go to a school that has 1100 students, on average ten students at that school would have ASDs. About four times as many boys have ASDs as girls, so at the school that has ten students with ASDs, on average eight of those ten ASD students would be boys.

Another question you may have is "What are the differences between people who have ASDs and those who do not (the NTs)?" The major difference is that people with ASDs have difficulty understanding and getting along with others. You may know a person with a reading disability. This means that compared with other people, that person has difficulty with reading and needs extra help. We could call having an ASD a social disability. Compared with others (the NTs), people with ASDs may have trouble making and keeping friends or just may not be as interested in having friends. They may not understand other people's thoughts and feelings very well, and they may have difficulty with understanding certain social clues such as facial expressions and personal space. People with ASDs may have very strong interests compared with NTs. They also may find it particularly hard when things change. The ASD person may want to do things in a certain order and in the same way every time.

There are people with ASDs who cannot talk or who were slow at learning to talk when they were small children. Others talk in unusual ways. For instance, some ASD children sound like "little professors" when they talk because they use so many big words. People with ASDs may not be good at pretending and instead may focus on facts and figures. People with ASDs may talk a lot about their special interests and may not be the best at giving other people their turn to talk. In the remaining chapters of this book, we will go over these differences in more depth and provide suggestions about how to handle any differences that concern you.

You may also wonder how people find out that they have an ASD. When we find out that someone has an ASD we say they have been diagnosed. When large differences are noticed by the parents of a young child, the child may be diagnosed with the ASD at that time. The child will be seen by a medical doctor and by other specialists, such as psychologists or social workers who have special knowledge about ASDs and other types of disorders. However, when there are only small to medium differences it can take many years before someone is diagnosed with an ASD. Some people are not diagnosed until they are teenagers or adults. Until about the mid 1990s, the children and adults who had small to medium differences were not diagnosed as having an ASD. They might have been described as different, quirky, unique, eccentric, loners, or odd. Over the past few years, we have figured out that some of these quirky or odd people have mild ASDs. Some adults find this out about themselves through their own research. Others do not find it out until another family member is diagnosed, and then they realize that they have some of the same issues. As a counselor, I have seen many parents realize that they have ASDs when one of their own children is diagnosed with an ASD.

This leads to another question that could be on your mind as a reader, and that is "Do I have an ASD?" Because ASDs can run in families as we discussed before, some children and teens who have a parent with an ASD will have an ASD themselves. If that is the case for you, it may have already been diagnosed. However, if you and your parents feel that there is a chance that you have an ASD but it has not already been diagnosed, your parents can talk to your doctor to see if it would be helpful to get tested. Most children and teens whose parents have ASDs are NTs (that is, they do not have ASDs). My sister and I are NTs but we do have other family members who have been diagnosed with ASDs.

There are currently several terms used to describe ASDs, but scientists are working on a new plan to change them all to "Autism Spectrum Disorder" in 2013. For now, though, you will hear other terms including autism, Autistic Disorder, Asperger's Syndrome, or even the very long name Pervasive Developmental Disorder, Not Otherwise Specified (abbreviated PDD.NOS). The important thing to know is that no matter which exact term is used, the ASDs have a lot in common. We will be learning more about the things they have in common in the remaining chapters.

One final thing is important to understand. Hundreds of thousands of people have ASDs, but they are not all alike. Although I will be describing the things they have in common in this book, there are more ways that people with ASDs are different than each other than ways they are alike. For instance, many hundreds of thousands of people also have diabetes. We could read a book about what people with diabetes have in common and learn about the problems they have with their blood sugar and their insulin production. By doing that we could get a better idea of what life is like for people with diabetes. We could learn ways to support a loved one who has diabetes, and we could learn to better understand the special problems they face. However, if we met a person with diabetes we would not think of the diabetes as the most important thing about them. The same is true of ASDs. The fact that someone has an ASD is just one piece of information about that person. We can get an idea of what life is like for people with ASDs. We can learn ways to support a loved one who has an ASD, and we can learn to better understand the special problems they face. However, the fact that our loved one has an ASD is not the most important thing about him or her. Each person with an ASD is a unique and wonderful human being with amazing potential—just like you!

There are things you can do to better understand your ASD parent. Have your parent fill out the first part of the worksheet below and then share it with you, so you can learn about your parent and about what he or she thinks is important. Then you can fill out the last part about yourself and share it with your family.

Parent section

Here is how I learned that I have an ASD:

☐ Another family member was diagnosed with an ASD and then I realized I might have one too. The other family member is:

_____

☐ I learned about ASDs by: _____ and then I realized I might have one too.

☐ Someone (_____) told me they thought I had an ASD.

☐ I went to a doctor or other specialist to see if I had an ASD.

☐ Other: _____

I was diagnosed with the following ASD (circle one): autism or Autistic Disorder, Asperger's Syndrome, PDD.NOS (Pervasive Development Disorder, Not Otherwise Specified), autism spectrum disorder.

The year that I was diagnosed was: _____

I had these feelings about being diagnosed with an ASD:

Relieved   Confused   Embarrassed   Angry   Sad   Worried

Other: _____

Here are other things about me that I think are important.

This is where I grew up: _____

_____

This is where I went to school: _____

These are a few important parts of my life story: _____

_____

_____

These are my favorite ways to spend free time: _____

_____

Here are some of the best things about me: _____

_____

_____

_____

Here are some of the problems I have at times: _____

_____

_____

_____

My favorite vacation was: _____

_____

I would like to accomplish these goals in my future: _____

_____

_____

_____

Section for the child or teen

☐ I am an NT (neurotypical).

☐ I am not sure if I have an ASD or if I am an NT.

☐ I have been diagnosed with the following ASD (circle one): autism or Autistic Disorder, Asperger's Syndrome, PDD.NOS (Pervasive Development Disorder, Not Otherwise Specified), autism spectrum disorder.

The year that I was diagnosed was: _____

I had these feelings about being diagnosed with an ASD:

   Relieved   Confused   Embarrassed   Angry   Sad   Worried

Other: _____

29

Chapter 4

Social Activities and Parties

When NT children or teens think of having their own birthday parties, they may think of the presents they hope to receive. If they are attending a friend's party, they may think of the present they will choose for their friend. They could be excited about the food and the birthday cake. Perhaps they hope to listen to music or play party games. The NT children and teens may feel nervous about meeting new people at the party, but most of the time their experience will tell them that the new people will like them and they might become friends.

What would it be like for ASD children and teens who had bad experiences at parties? What if they often received presents that were completely uninteresting to them? What if the ASD child only liked chocolate cake with chocolate frosting and instead carrot cake with vanilla frosting was served? What if the noise level at parties made these children and teens feel very stressed, so that they then got upset or left, leading the other guests to get mad at them for causing a problem? What if the ASD children wanted so badly to win at the games that when they lost they were devastated and were not able to have a good time after that? What would it be like for the children who talked for ten minutes about a special interest such as marine animals or astronomy and then the other kids teased them and called them nerds?

People with ASDs often have these kinds of experiences at social activities such as parties, family reunions, and special events. Therefore it is possible that your ASD parent finds social activities either uninteresting or stressful. Your parent might choose not to attend social activities or, if he or she does attend, may not want to socialize very much. ASD adults who do attend social activities may read a book or use their laptop instead of spending time talking with people. At social activities there is often "small talk" that people use to get to know each other, when they talk about "small" things such as the weather, or traffic, or vacation plans. People with ASDs may find this kind of small talk meaningless and boring. They may prefer to talk about something that they know a lot about (such as their special interest, which we will discuss in Chapter 6), but they may not be able to find anyone who shares that interest. The room may be noisy with loud music playing, and ASD adults may prefer it when a room is quiet and orderly. They might feel more comfortable socializing only with their own family or with very close friends. They may prefer doing an activity they particularly enjoy such as playing a video game or a board game, or going to an event such as a movie or a play that does not involve much socializing.

When I was a child, my father did not attend social activities very often even if the activities were important to the rest of us. He definitely did not like small talk, and he did not like being with people outside of the family all that much. If he did go to a social activity, he would bring a book to read no matter where we went (remember this was before there were laptops and cell phones). He would even read his book at the dinner table, when the rest of us were talking about the day. When my mother retired, he did not go to her retirement dinner because he did not have any interest in socializing with the other people who would be attending, even though my mother had worked with those people for years.

As a counselor, when I work with ASD adults in a group activity or in a class, they may be particularly quiet and may appear shy or bored. Sometimes they talk a lot about a particular topic of special interest to them (you will read more on this in the next two chapters). The ASD adults may sit at the back of the class and may not get to know the other group members very quickly. They may not stay and visit with me or other adults after class.

So, what about you? Has it ever been difficult for you if your ASD parent did not attend an important social activity with you? Have you ever been embarrassed if your ASD parent sat in the hall while the other adults talked and laughed? Has anyone ever said they thought your ASD parent was rude because of how he or she acted at a social activity? When I was young my father rarely attended my special events such as my Girl Scout award dinners or the parades in which I marched. I was sad that my father was not there. I would feel jealous when I saw other fathers at these special events. Children I know who have ASD parents tell me they sometimes feel sad or embarrassed by things that happen at social get-togethers, such as if their parent leaves the room or acts in a way that others think is rude.

Complete this chapter's worksheet with your family so you can all learn about each other and develop new skills to handle social activities and parties.

Rate how you much you enjoy social activities or parties on a scale of 0 to 10:

    0   1   2   3   4   5   6   7   8   9   10

    I don't enjoy   I love
    them at all   them

Have your ASD parent rate how he or she enjoys social activities or parties on a scale of 0 to 10:

    0   1   2   3   4   5   6   7   8   9   10

    I don't enjoy   I love
    them at all   them

If you have other family members that you would like to rate, add their details at the bottom of the page.

Name of person: _____ Rating: _____

Name of person: _____ Rating: _____

If any family members have a low rating, have them check off the ways that they handle social activities.

☐ Sometimes I choose not to go.

☐ I bring things with me to do: _____

_____

☐ I only go if I have a friend who will be there with me.

☐ I only like to attend certain social activities. The social activities I like to attend are: _____

_____

☐ Other ways I handle social activities: _____

_____

_____

Circle the feelings you have had if there has been difficulty about your parent attending social activities with you:

Sad   Angry   Hurt   Embarrassed

Confused   Guilty

Other: _____

Go through the following list of problem-solving skills together and check the ones you want to try:

☐ If a particular activity is very important to me, I can explain why it is important and ask my parent to please come with me.

☐ I can find someone else to attend important social activities with me.

☐ We can find social activities that we both like and enjoy.

Some ideas are: _____

_____

☐ We can find ways to compromise about social activities, such as going for a shorter time, or going less often.

☐ I can work on accepting that my parent and I feel differently about social activities. I can think about the other things I like about my parent, such as: _____

_____

_____

_____

_____

Chapter 5

Conversations and Figures of Speech

When NT children and teens talk to friends, they may take turns talking about topics they both enjoy. Occasionally they may change the subject quickly, but when they do, they usually know to warn the other person first. For instance, they might say, "I know this is random, but ___" or "I know I'm changing the subject, but ___." NT children and teens know if they talk too long without giving their friend a turn that the friend will get bored or frustrated. They also probably know that when someone says, "You must be pulling my leg," then the person thinks he or she is being told something that is not true. If they hear the metaphor "She had ants in her pants" they realize that this is just another way of saying that she was very wriggly. If they hear a simile, such as "That tree was as tall as a skyscraper!" in all likelihood they know it is just a way of saying that the tree was very tall. NT children and teens are also able to change the meaning of the words they say by changing their tone of voice.

What is it like for the ASD children and teens who do not understand the back and forth of a conversation and blurt things out randomly? What happens when they do not catch the signals that someone is bored? Would they feel confused if someone said, "You must be pulling my leg" when they knew they were not touching the person's leg? Is there a chance they would feel irritated if they read a metaphor that said, "She had ants in her pants" when they knew that there were no actual bugs in her clothes? Would they argue with a friend if they heard him or her use the simile "That tree is as tall as a skyscraper!" if they knew that the tree was not nearly as tall as a real skyscraper? What if they even had extra trouble understanding the phrase since the word "skyscraper" is itself a metaphor? What would it be like for children to get teased for having a "boring" voice but then not know what to do to make their voice sound "interesting"? ASD children and teens sometimes work with speech therapists (also called speech "pathologists") to learn how to fix these types of problems.

People who have ASDs may have these problems with conversations and figures of speech. They may not be good at the flow of a conversation and may say things at odd times. They might talk too much about their special interest. They are known to have the tendency to "go on and on" about certain subjects and not notice that others are not as interested as they are in what they are talking about. They might not understand metaphors, similes, or analogies, and they may speak in a monotone voice ("mono" means one, so "monotone" means using only one tone in the voice).

When I was a child, my father usually did not talk much to other people. When other people tried to talk to him, he would not keep the conversation going back and forth, unless the topic was one of his special interests. He would say, "Squirrels are more interesting than people!" as his way of commenting on this issue. He would ask other people if they played chess, even when that was not a relevant part of the conversation. He also had a habit of swearing frequently if something upset him.

In counseling, the counselor and clients often spend a few minutes discussing how things are going to get relaxed and comfortable before they get down to the business of the therapy session. However, ASD adults may not ask me about how things have been going since how I am doing is not technically related to the actual purpose of our appointment, which is specifically about how they have been doing. They frequently will walk ahead of me down the hall to my office, rather than walking and talking with me as an NT client might.

What about you? Have you ever noticed any of these differences when your ASD parent is talking? Have there ever been times when you felt embarrassed because your ASD parent was talking too much about his or her own interests? When I was a child, I would feel self-conscious when my father swore in front of other people and then did not apologize to them or even notice their bad reactions to his language. Children with ASD parents sometimes tell me that they feel their parents do not really listen to them, because they do not get their turn to talk as often as they would like.

Complete this worksheet with your family so you can all learn about each other and develop new skills to handle problems with conversations and figures of speech.

Below are listed different conversation problems. First check to see if you have any of the problems. Then have your ASD parent and other family members check to see if they have any of the problems. It can be helpful for everyone in the family to look over the ratings and mark problems that they observe, because there are times when people are not aware that they do these things.

Conversation problems	You	Your ASD parent	Other family members
Changing topics too quickly			
Talking too much and not giving turns			
Not talking enough			
Not understanding figures of speech			
Not enjoying "small talk"			
Talking in a monotone voice			
Other:			

Circle the feelings you have when your ASD parent has these kinds of conversation problems:

Sad   Angry   Hurt   Embarrassed   Confused   Guilty

Other: _____

Go through the following list of problem-solving skills together and check the ones you want to try:

☐ When someone changes the topic of conversation too quickly, a plan could be set up to get a signal from someone else in the family.

☐ When someone is going to change the topic of conversation, he or she could learn to give a warning, such as, "I know I'm changing the topic, but there is something I really want to tell you."

☐ When someone talks too much and does not let other people have their turn, he or she could let others know by saying something like: "Sometimes I talk too much about things I am really interested in. When I am talking too much, please let me know."

☐ When someone talks too much, he or she could work on learning the clues that show when someone is bored (such as a "blank," confused, or irritated look on the person's face, or the person looking away or checking the time) and could learn to stop talking when he or she sees those clues.

☐ When someone does not talk enough, others can try to ask more detailed questions, such as, "What did you do this morning?" instead of more general questions, such as, "How are you doing?"

☐ When someone does not talk enough, he or she can make an effort to say at least two or three things in every conversation to make other people feel more comfortable.

☐ When someone is not sure what a certain figure of speech means, he or she can say, "I'm not too great with figures of speech. Can you say that another way?"

☐ When someone is not sure what a certain figure of speech means, he or she could look up the meaning in a dictionary of idioms.

☐ When someone does not like small talk, he or she can learn to say, "I'm sorry. I really don't enjoy small talk. Please don't take it personally."

☐ When someone does not like small talk, he or she can learn a few things to say in these kinds of situations to make other people feel more comfortable.

Chapter 6

Special Interests

NT children and teens generally have special interests, activities, and hobbies that are important to them. They may like sports, hiking, or dance. They may like to listen to music, play an instrument, or sing. They may enjoy certain television shows or movies, and they may look forward to the nights when they can watch their favorite shows. They might have hobbies such as doing puzzles or making crafts. They may be artists or actors. Many NT children and teens like gaming or using their computers. They may work on their hobbies whenever they get some free time and may look forward to doing their favorite activities on the weekends or during school vacations.

ASD children and teens may be so obsessed with their special interests, favorite activities, or hobbies that they cannot think about anything else. They may feel that they cannot stand it when they are not able to do their special interest, and then they may get in trouble for refusing to do other things such as their homework or chores. They may have trouble letting go of a special interest that others their age have outgrown. What would it be like for an ASD child in sixth grade who still enjoyed an activity that had been popular in third grade and was teased because the other kids at school now thought that game was babyish? ASD children and teens may know a great deal about their special interest, and they may be able to tell you all kinds of facts and figures about it. Their interest may be one that many other people share (such as dinosaurs or gaming or baseball) or it may be one that is not shared by that many others (such as types of snails or license plates).

People with ASDs generally continue to have very strong special interests right into adulthood. Sometimes ASD adults continue interests they developed when they were children, such as studying astronomy or reading fantasy books. At other times they might develop a new interest, such as online computer gaming or geo-caching (a kind of high-tech treasure hunt). The chances are they spend quite a bit of time and money doing things related to their special interest. A person whose special interest is studying astronomy might collect books about astronomy, have many different telescopes for looking at the night sky, read astronomy blogs and websites, go to planetariums, attend meetings with amateur astronomers, and set his or her work schedule around star or planet sightings. Even if the person does not normally enjoy socializing, he or she might enjoy being around astronomers in order to talk about astronomy. Some ASD adults do advanced studies in their special interest, and they may end up with a job in that field. There are times when people with ASDs are so involved with their special interest that they do not get other things done that are important to their job or their family.

When I was a child, my father had several special interests over those years, including chess, birdwatching, food, literature, classical music, tennis, and following politics. His all-time favorite special interest was chess. He had one of the largest libraries of chess books and magazines in the United States. The books and magazines were in many different languages including German, Russian, French, Serbo-Croat, and Bulgarian. He would then study those other languages so that he could read the books and magazines. He ran chess clubs and wrote weekly chess columns for newspapers. He wrote a chess column for the *Boston Herald* for over 40 years. Whenever he met new people, he would ask them if they played chess because he was always hoping to find new chess partners.

When I am counseling adults with ASDs, I have to be careful to try to find a balance between hearing the latest news about their special interest and accomplishing the task we are supposed to be working on in our therapy session. However, if I have a question about a particular topic, and I know an adult with an ASD who has a special interest in that area, I know that I might be able to go to that person to get an answer to my question because he or she is likely to be an expert.

What has this been like for you? Does your ASD parent have a special interest? Is it an interest that you enjoy also or is it something that causes you some stress? When I was in elementary school, I enjoyed participating in my father's special interests. He taught me how to play chess, and I would play in children's chess tournaments that he organized. We would also go birdwatching together and discuss politics when we watched the news on television. When I got older, I lost interest in chess and birdwatching. Then it was difficult because I felt that my father was not as interested in me since I did not want to play chess with him or go for drives to look for birds.

I have known children who are frustrated because they do not get as much time as they would like with their ASD parents because of their parents' special interests.

Complete this worksheet with your family so you can all learn about each other and develop new skills to handle any problems connected to special interests.

Write down your favorite activity or interest: _____

Rate your level of interest in your favorite activity on a scale of 0 to 10:

| 0 | 1 | 2 | 3 | 4 | 5 | 6 | 7 | 8 | 9 | 10 |

Just a little   I'm obsessed
interested   by it!

Have your ASD parent write down his or her favorite activity:

_____

Then have your parent rate the level of his or her interest on the same scale of 0 to 10:

| 0 | 1 | 2 | 3 | 4 | 5 | 6 | 7 | 8 | 9 | 10 |

Just a little   I'm obsessed
interested   by it!

If you have other family members, get their ratings.

Name	Favorite activity	Interest level on scale of 1-10

Are there any ways that these special interests have been positive for your family?

☐ We all enjoy doing this special interest together:

_____

☐ We have made money with this special interest:

_____

☐ We have learned a lot from this special interest:

_____

☐ Other ways it has been positive: _____

_____

Circle the feelings you have when your parent is spending time on his or her special interest:

Sad   Angry   Happy   Hurt   Jealous   Confused

Other: _____

Go through the following list of problem-solving skills together and check the ones you want to try:

☐ My parent and I can spend more time doing one of the interests that we both enjoy.

Here is how we could do that together: _____

_____

☐ My parent has an interest I would like to learn more about:

_____

Here is how we could do that together: _____

_____

☐ My parent and I would like to develop a new interest together.

Here is how we could do that together: _____

_____

☐ I have an interest my parent would like to learn more about:

_____

Here is how we could do that together: _____

_____

☐ I can ask my parent to spend more time with me. Here is how I could talk about it:

When you spend a lot of time on your special interest, I feel

_____ (name your feeling), because

_____ .

I wish you would: _____ .

Chapter 7

Understanding Others

When you are doing things with your friends or your family, there may be times when each person wants something different. If you are ordering a pizza as a family, you may want pepperoni, but your sister, the vegetarian, wants onions and mushrooms, your father, who is trying to lose weight, wants a "light" version, and your brother, the cheese lover, wants extra cheese. Even though NT children and teens may find it annoying to work out a compromise that each person in the family can accept, they understand that each person has a different idea of what makes the best pizza. When a friend loses his or her iPod, NT children or teens will have a good idea of how the friend is feeling because they know what their friend is like and how important the iPod is to him or her. Additionally, if they see their parents having a disagreement, they might have a fairly good guess about how their parents are feeling towards each other at such a moment. This is because over time NT children and teens have learned how the people they know best see the world. When we can understand other people's thoughts, plans, and feelings then it is easier to get along with others and to predict or imagine what might happen next. We use the metaphor "being in someone else's shoes" to explain what happens when we try to see things from another person's point of view. Additionally, NT children and teens are able to reflect on and talk about their own thoughts, plans, and feelings, and they know how to be flexible in their thinking. Being flexible in this way does not mean that they can touch their toes! It means they can think about something in a number of different ways rather than just in one exact or rigid way.

What is it like for ASD children and teens who are not able to "be in someone else's shoes" because their brains are not wired to allow them to think in that way? What is it like when they do not understand another person's thoughts, plans, or feelings? What is it like for ASD children and teens when they find it difficult to reflect on and talk about their own thoughts, plans, and feelings? People may get mad at them and think they are lying when they truthfully answer, "I don't know" to questions about their feelings. ASD children and teens may find the process of deciding on the pizza more than just a little annoying, because it may not make sense to them that someone else could want vegetables when they want pepperoni. They also may not have any idea how their friend felt when that iPod was lost. They may not have been able to guess what their mother and father were thinking about each other during the disagreement. This type of problem has been called "mindblindness." This means that people with ASDs have extra trouble guessing (that is, they are "blind to") what is going on in other people's minds. This can lead to them feeling confused and stressed about what is going on for others.

ASD adults may not be very expressive about their own feelings, and they may find it more natural and comfortable to talk about the facts of a situation than about the feelings of the people involved in the situation. They also may not show much interest in or understanding of other people's feelings. The ability to understand and share the feelings of another is called having empathy. If your parent is not skilled at understanding and sharing your feelings, it can be said that your parent is not very empathetic.

When I was a child, my father had a habit of talking negatively about people who had different opinions than his. He placed a lot of importance on being smart, and he often said he did not understand it when someone he thought was smart had an opinion different than his own. He did not show much concern about hurting others' feelings. When I was a teenager and began to think differently than he did about things (in the way that most teenagers do), he would get mad at me rather than trying to understand how I was seeing the world.

When I am counseling ASD parents, they find it particularly difficult to work on the skill of what counselors call "validation." Validation is when you try to show someone else that you understand how they think and feel, even if you do not agree. This can be very hard to do if your brain is wired to make it hard to see things from another's point of view. Many ASD parents find it hard to be in counseling with their children, because counseling involves talking about feelings.

How does this go in your family? Does your ASD parent find it difficult to understand different points of view (mindblindness)? Does your ASD parent have trouble showing empathy for you (remember, empathy means understanding and sharing your feelings)? Do you ever find this difficult? When I was little I was worried that my father thought I was stupid, since he talked so much about other people being stupid. Children tell me that their ASD parents do not understand their feelings or their thoughts well, especially when their opinions on a topic are different than their ASD parent's opinion. ASD adults often find partners who are very skilled at understanding other people's thoughts, plans, and feelings. This way the person who has strong skills can help the partner who has weak skills. This happened in my family, since my mother was a nurse by profession, and she was very caring and empathetic.

Complete this worksheet with your family so you can all learn about each other and develop new skills to handle problems with understanding others.

Rate how well you understand other people's thoughts, plans, and feelings on a scale of 0 to 10:

0   1   2   3   4   5   6   7   8   9   10

One of   One of
my weak   my strong
points   points

Have your ASD parent rate how well he or she understands other people's thoughts, plans, and feelings on a scale of 1 to 10:

0   1   2   3   4   5   6   7   8   9   10

One of   One of
my weak   my strong
points   points

If you have other family members, get their ratings.

Name of person: _____ Rating: _____

Name of person: _____ Rating: _____

Circle the feelings you have when your parent is not understanding your thoughts, plans, or feelings:

Sad   Angry   Worried   Confused

Disappointed   Hurt

Other: _____

Go through the following list of problem-solving skills together and check the ones you want to try:

☐ When I feel my parent does not understand my thoughts, plans, or feelings, I can try to explain them carefully. For instance, I can use an "I message," which goes like this:

When_____(describe

the behavior or situation), I feel _____

(the name of my feeling), because_____.

I wish_____

_____.

☐ When I feel my parent does not understand my thoughts, plans, or feelings, my parent can try to use the skill of "validation." This means my parent would listen carefully when I explain my thoughts and feelings and then explain how my thoughts and feelings make sense even if he or she does not agree. After listening to me explain, my parent could say, "It sounds like you think _____. Have I got that right? Is there anything else you would like me to understand about how you think and feel?" Keep in mind, as we said above, that learning to use the skill of validation can be especially hard for people with ASDs.

Chapter 8

Body Language

There are many ways in which we communicate what we think and feel. We use words to send one part of the message. We also use facial expressions to send another part of the message. Our facial expressions show that we are happy, sad, confused, or angry. We use gestures to send part of our message, such as nodding or shaking our heads for yes or no, waving our hands as a greeting when we see a friend, rubbing our hands together to show we are looking forward to something, giving a thumbs-up to show we like something, or shaking a finger at someone to show we do not like something. We use our posture to send another part of the message. Think of the different message we get if we see a friend who is sitting slumped in a chair holding her head in her hands, compared with the message we get when we see a friend who is sitting up straight, smiling, and looking at us. We also use our eyes to send part of the message. We send a different message when we make eye contact with a friend than when we look at the floor. Making eye contact usually means we are interested in our friend, while looking at the floor might indicate we are not interested. A message is also sent by how close we stand to others. We tend to stand closer to people who are good friends and farther away from people we do not know well. We use the term "body language" to describe any of these messages we send with our bodies. Social scientists, who study how people communicate, have found that at least half of a message is sent with our body language alone, while the rest of the message is sent with our words. It is also important to note that different cultures use body language differently.

We might think of sending messages between people as similar to using two radio stations at the same time. We use one radio station to send the first part of the message, the words, and the other radio station to send the second part of the message, the body language. NTs are able to tune to both radio stations at the same time, and therefore they send and receive the whole message: the words and the body language. ASD children and teens may only tune to the first radio station, the one that sends and receives the words. They may have trouble tuning to the second radio station that sends and receives the body language. What would it be like to miss important parts of almost every message? What would it be like to be misunderstood regularly? ASD children and teens may feel frustrated when others think they "meant" something by the fact that they were not making eye contact or because they had a certain expression on their face.

People with ASDs often do not use a large number of facial expressions and gestures. They may not use much eye contact, recognize others' need for personal space, or notice the meaning behind someone's posture. Sometimes ASD children and teens go to social skills groups to learn to understand and use body language better. Some people with ASDs also have unusual habits such as rocking or pacing, putting things in their mouths, tapping their fingers, or flapping their arms. These habits are another way in which body language is different for people with ASDs because NTs often find those ASD habits annoying. However, these habits can be difficult for people with ASDs to change because they are caused by how their brains are wired.

When I was a child, my father did not show much physical affection. That is, he did not show that he cared for us with his body language. He would say the words "I love you" but he did not give many hugs or kisses, or use other gestures of affection. He also did not have many different facial expressions. He could look happy or angry and he did make eye contact, but sometimes it felt like he was staring because he did not look away as quickly as other people would.

When I am counseling adults with ASDs, one of the first things I notice is that they may not show many facial expressions. In fact, that is one of the differences that may lead me to wonder if someone has an ASD. Instead, they often look serious no matter what subject we are discussing. I notice that ASD adults may not make much eye contact. I have learned to ask more questions about what adults with ASDs are thinking and feeling, so that I do not take the wrong message from their body language (such as assuming they are not listening because they are not making eye contact, or assuming they are angry because of a serious facial expression).

What about you? Have you ever been confused by getting different messages from your ASD parent's words and from his or her body language? Has your ASD parent ever misunderstood you because he or she was not tuning into the message you were sending with your body language? Have your friends ever wondered why your ASD parent does not make eye contact? When I was a child, I sometimes mistakenly thought my father was angry because of the serious look on his face. Children tell me they wish that their ASD parents would look at them more because they are worried that the lack of eye contact means that their parent is not interested in them.

Complete this worksheet with your family so you can all learn about each other and develop new skills to handle body language problems.

Rate how well you send and receive body language messages on a scale of 0 to 10:

0   1   2   3   4   5   6   7   8   9   10

One of   One of
my weak   my strong
points   points

Have your ASD parent rate how well he or she sends and receives body language messages on a scale of 0 to 10:

0   1   2   3   4   5   6   7   8   9   10

One of   One of
my weak   my strong
points   points

If you have other family members, get their ratings.

Name of person: _____ Rating: _____

Name of person: _____ Rating: _____

Circle the feelings you have when your parent is not sending or receiving the body language messages very well:

Sad   Angry   Worried   Confused

Disappointed   Hurt

Other: _____

Go through the following list of problem-solving skills together and check the ones you want to try:

☐ I can learn to check with my parent about the message he or she is sending, to make sure that I am receiving the correct one. I can learn to say, "I think you mean _____. Have I got that right?"

☐ My parent can learn to check with me about my message, to make sure that the "whole" message I sent was received. He or she can learn to say, "I think you mean _____. Have I got that right?"

☐ My parent can read a book about body language to learn more about tuning into body language messages.

☐ If my parent has any movements that have bothered me in the past, I can learn to accept that they are caused by how my parent's brain is wired.

Chapter 9

Emotions

While children and teens are growing up and maturing they are learning how to handle their feelings. A very interesting part of being human is that we have so many different feelings, such as anger, sadness, fear, and happiness, to name just a few. Then, to make it even more interesting, different situations lead different people to have different feelings! One person might feel happy to get to go on a boat, while another might feel scared in the same situation. One person might find that the idea of the family getting a new video game makes them angry while another finds it makes them happy. For instance, a parent who does not like their children to spend time gaming might feel angry, while the son or daughter who loves gaming might be happy. We can also notice another difference. People of different ages are different in how well they can handle their feelings. If a two-year-old girl is disappointed about not getting a candy bar at the store, she might throw herself on the floor and have a temper tantrum before forgetting about it. If a 12-year-old girl is disappointed about not getting a candy bar at the store, she might say, "Oh well" before forgetting about it.

Children and teens with ASDs may find it harder to learn how to handle their feelings because there are ways in which their feelings are different than those of NTs. They may find it harder to use words to explain their feelings. Some people with ASDs have very strong, intense feelings about both small and large situations. Other people with ASDs may show very little feeling at all. Additionally, because people with ASDs have trouble with being able to "be in someone else's shoes," it can be harder for them to understand that they are responsible for their own feelings and so instead they may think that other people cause their feelings.

Many NT and ASD people have special problems with their feelings. These special problems are called "disorders," just like autism is a type of disorder. If some people get scared or worried a lot more than others, and these fears cause problems in their lives, they may have an anxiety disorder. If some people get sad or angry a lot more than others, and this amount of sadness or anger is causing problems in their lives, they may have depression. If some people find their feelings go up and down a lot, and these mood swings cause problems in their lives, they may have Bipolar Disorder (which means their moods go between two extremes, or "poles"). If some people are less able to pay attention than others, and are more hyper (hyperactive) than others, and these issues are causing problems in their lives, they may have Attention Deficit Hyperactivity Disorder (ADHD). These kinds of disorders are diagnosed by doctors or counselors. You probably know people with these kinds of emotional problems, and you may even have one yourself. People with ASDs are somewhat more likely than NTs to have one of these emotional problems. However, keep in mind that many NTs have these emotional problems, and many people with ASDs do not have them. People with one of these emotional problems may take medication, see a counselor, or learn other ways of making changes so they can learn to feel better.

When I was growing up, my father had trouble handling his anger. When he got angry, he would yell and swear, and pace around the house. He also had trouble handling his worries. He would get very worried when he was going to be in a chess tournament and he complained about not being able to sleep on the nights before tournaments. He probably had an anxiety disorder, but there was not much help available then for people who had trouble with their worries.

ASD adults talk to me about having trouble handling their anger. They also tell me about problems with mood swings, sadness, and worry. They sometimes find it harder to get help than NT adults, because not as many counselors know how to help ASD adults. As everyone learns more about ASDs, counselors and doctors included, people with ASDs will be able to get more help for their emotional problems.

Children and teens who have ASD parents sometimes talk to me about their parents getting overly angry with them. This may scare them, or it may lead to them to getting mad in return. One of the common goals in counseling when someone has an anger problem is to work out a safety plan for everyone. In a safety plan everyone stays away from each other in different rooms for a little while, and the angry person follows steps to calm down. When I was a child I used to be scared of my father when he got angry, and I would hide in my bedroom at those times. I also tried to be careful not to do things that might make him mad, because I did not realize until I was older that he was responsible for his own feelings and that his anger was not my fault.

Complete this worksheet with your family so you can all learn about each other and develop new skills to handle emotional problems.

Rate how well you handle your feelings on a scale of 0 to 10:

0   1   2   3   4   5   6   7   8   9   10

One of
my weak
points

One of
my strong
points

Have your ASD parent rate how well he or she handles feelings on a scale of 0 to 10:

0   1   2   3   4   5   6   7   8   9   10

One of
my weak
points

One of
my strong
points

If you have other family members, get their ratings.

Name of person: _____ Rating: _____

Name of person: _____ Rating: _____

Circle the emotions you have when a family member has problems with his or her feelings (such as being overly worried, angry, or sad):

Embarrassed   Sad   Angry   Worried

Confused   Disappointed   Hurt

Other: _____

Go through the following list of problem-solving skills together and check the ones you want to try.

If someone in my family has strong feelings that are causing problems, he or she can:

☐ see a doctor or counselor for help

☐ read a book or information on the internet to get help

☐ talk to clergy at our place of worship for advice

☐ take better care of his or her feelings by taking care of the body (such as getting more exercise or more sleep, or eating better)

☐ make some changes in the family schedule to reduce stress (such as: _____)

☐ go to a support group or spend more time with friends to get support.

Chapter 10

Learning and Organizing

When NT children and teens are asked to write a summary of a story at school, or to explain the main point of a history lesson, they are usually able to do so in a few sentences. They try to learn how to keep their backpacks and school work organized, and to keep track of their homework assignments. They know that if they have to turn in a book report in three weeks they must plan it out. For instance, they may read the book over the first two weeks, then write a draft of the book report, make corrections, and then turn in the final report when it is due. They have also learned to bring home their jackets from school each day, and to tell their parents about signing forms for upcoming field trips. They have been learning to understand words for abstract ideas (things you cannot see or touch, such as "freedom" and "friendship") and words for concrete items (things you can see or touch, such as "pizza" or "dog"). They usually remember the names of their friends and teachers. NT children are usually able to tell the time by early in elementary school. They generally care about their appearance, so they make sure to shower, wear clean clothes that are in fashion, and style their hair.

What do you think it is like for ASD children and teens when they feel they have to tell every detail of the book they have read even if they have been asked to write just a summary? What if they tried hard to keep their desks and backpacks organized but still frequently lost their homework and others kept getting mad at them about it? What would they be feeling if they kept losing other important things, such as their MP3 players or their lunch money? What if they found it hard to understand abstract words because they cannot see, hear, or touch those abstract ideas? What if appearance seemed very unimportant to them compared with the more meaningful things in life, so they did not worry about whether their clothes were in fashion, or what their hair looked like, and then they were teased about their appearance? What would it be like for them if they could rarely remember the names of the other children or of their teachers, or had trouble understanding time? These are some of the experiences of children and teens with ASDs.

Adults with ASDs continue to have these issues. They often have trouble staying organized and remembering the day's schedule, especially when it is different than the usual routine. Interestingly enough, they may do exceptionally well remembering facts and events that are connected to their special interest but then have more trouble with day-to-day things such as remembering to get milk on the way home from work, or the names of their children's friends. In this way we could think of adults with ASDs as similar to the stereotype of the "absent-minded professor." It is also important to mention that not all adults with ASDs are disorganized. Instead, some may be very orderly and want everything done in just a certain way (you can read more on this in Chapter 12). Adults with ASDs often do not care much about hygiene, clothing fashions, or hairstyles, and they may think of such things as silly or trivial. They often do better with understanding concrete details and facts and figures rather than abstract ideas or main points. Adults with ASDs might not know how to respond to certain kinds of questions appropriately. For instance, when asked "How was your vacation?" they might give too much detail about everything they did and take a long time to answer the question, rather than just give the main point of the vacation (such as "We stayed in a condo by the beach and really enjoyed swimming in the water every day and visiting the grandparents"). They might not realize that most people would expect this kind of brief summary of a trip.

My father definitely fit the stereotype of the absent-minded professor, and he was even a teacher by profession! He could remember all the moves of hundreds of different chess games, but he could not remember to do an errand on his way home from school. If he did stop at the store at my mother's request, he would get the snacks he liked but forget the items the rest of us needed. He was always neat and clean, but he wore the same style of clothing to work for 30 years and thought it was silly when people suggested he try wearing a shirt color other than white for a change.

As a counselor, when I meet adults with ASDs, they are usually not the best at organizing their family's schedule. Often the spouse does the family scheduling. Their clothes may be rumpled and not very fashionable, and they may not look well groomed. When I teach things in counseling, I may give them a written list of their "therapy homework" to help them remember rather than expect them to remember it on their own.

What about you? Has there ever been any difficulty for you or for your family due to your ASD parent being disorganized? Have there been any problems about things getting lost? Have you ever been embarrassed because of your ASD parent's quirky or messy appearance? When I was a child, we used to tease my father about the everyday items he would forget to do. When I was a teenager, I felt embarrassed by the fact that my father's clothes were not in style. Children sometimes tell me they get frustrated about the things that their ASD parent forgets, such as their appointments with me!

Complete this worksheet with your family so you can all learn about each other and develop new skills to handle problems with learning and organizing.

Rate how organized you are on a scale of 0 to 10:

0   1   2   3   4   5   6   7   8   9   10

One of
my weak
points

One of
my strong
points

Have your ASD parent rate how organized he or she is on a scale of 0 to 10:

0   1   2   3   4   5   6   7   8   9   10

One of
my weak
points

One of
my strong
points

If you have other family members, get their ratings.

Name of person: _____ Rating: _____

Name of person: _____ Rating: _____

Circle the feelings you have when the family is disorganized:

Sad   Angry   Worried   Confused

Disappointed   Hurt

Other: _____

Rate how interested you are in clothing, fashion, and hairstyles on a scale of 0 to 10.

0   1   2   3   4   5   6   7   8   9   10

I am   I am very
not interested   interested
at all

Have your ASD parent rate how interested he or she is in clothing, fashion, and hairstyles on a scale of 0 to 10.

0   1   2   3   4   5   6   7   8   9   10

I am   I am very
not interested   interested
at all

If you have other family members, get their ratings.

Name of person: _____ Rating: _____

Name of person: _____ Rating: _____

Circle the feelings you have if your parent's appearance is quirky or messy:

Embarrassed   Sad   Angry   Worried

Confused   Disappointed

Other: _____

Go through the following list of problem-solving skills together and check the ones you want to try:

☐ We can try a new plan for staying organized, such as using a family calendar or planner (either a paper or a computerized one).

☐ We can set up family meetings once or twice a week to help our family stay organized.

☐ We can read a book on how to become better organized or get help from a counselor or other specialist.

☐ If there is a certain time when my parent's appearance will be particularly important to me, I can let him or her know ahead of time what the other parents will be likely to be wearing and why that event is special to me.

☐ A family member or a friend can be a fashion coach for my ASD parent and remind him or her about certain times when it would be best to get dressed up or get a haircut.

☐ I can work on accepting that my parent does not think that appearance is important.

Chapter 11

Humor and Imagination

Many NT children and teens enjoy hearing jokes and listening to funny stories. They may also be good at telling jokes and making sarcastic comments. NT children may enjoy acting out imaginative games and otherwise pretending that things are different than real life. Many games that children and teens play are based on ways to be funny or imaginative. Another thing that is based on being imaginative is writing fiction, and at school students regularly have to write fictional stories. Additionally, NT children have learned that sometimes people may use words in ways that are not literally true. If a friend says, "I'm so mad at Jacob—I could just strangle him!" NT children know this does not mean their friend is truly going to strangle Jacob, but that they are "just words" that show their friend is feeling angry with Jacob.

What do you think it is like for ASD children or teenagers who do not understand jokes very well? Will they feel confused or left out when everyone else is laughing at a joke that they do not understand? Even worse, imagine how they might feel if they misunderstand why everyone is laughing and think that they are being laughed at instead of the joke. What would it be like to "not get" sarcasm? Sarcasm can be hard to understand since it is a way of making a joke by saying the opposite of what is truly meant. What about the children who cannot think of anything to write about when their teacher asks them to write a story about the future, because it is hard for them to imagine something that has not yet happened? What is it like for children who think that people literally mean everything they say? Would that child be afraid for Jacob's safety when they heard the friend say she was so mad at Jacob that she wanted to strangle him?

ASD children and teens often have difficulty understanding humor. They also may have trouble with understanding imaginative ideas or playing pretend games. ASD adults may continue to miss the meaning of some jokes and may not be the best at telling jokes either. Telling a good joke often requires skills that people with ASDs lack, such as being able to use different tones of voice, making use of body language and facial expressions, and being able to understand different shades of meaning. They tend to be better at writing about details and facts than about imaginative ideas. Sometimes it will look as if children or teens with ASDs are very imaginative, because they might spend hours involved in fantasy role-playing games or acting out a scene from a movie such as *Star Wars*. However, when one looks carefully at these types of games, it can be seen that they are not imagining their own characters but instead are using ideas that have been created by the authors.

My father would start certain joke routines with his grandchildren when they were little and then continue it on for years, even when they were too grown up for that joke still to be funny to them. He had a habit of cocking his fingers like a gun and pretending to shoot at my son, who was four or five at the time. Back then, my son thought it was funny and would pretend to shoot back at him. However, now that son is 15 and he does not think it is funny any longer, but my father continues to do it as if nothing has changed.

When I am counseling people with ASDs, I try to be careful about my use of sarcasm so that my meaning is understood correctly. If I do use sarcasm, I am careful to give obvious hints that the words I am saying are the opposite of what I truly mean or I check for understanding afterwards. I also find that I end up teaching children and teens with ASDs about humor, such as helping them learn not to repeat jokes that could be offensive or that do not make much sense. Some of the ASD adults I know are very literal, and they tell me how much trouble they had in college classes when they had to write fiction or do other imaginative assignments.

What have you noticed about your ASD parent's humor and imagination? Is there sometimes confusion over the meaning of a joke? Have there been times when your parent took something too literally and got needlessly upset, because it was not "meant" in the way he or she took it? Some children have told me they get embarrassed by their ASD parent's poor sense of humor and the bad jokes he or she tells.

Complete this worksheet with your family so you can all learn about each other and develop new skills to handle problems relating to humor and imagination.

Below are listed problems relating to humor and imagination. First, mark whether you have any of the problems. Then, have your ASD parent and other family members do the same.

Problems with humor and imagination	You	Your ASD parent	Other family members
Taking things too literally			
Difficulty with creative writing			
Difficulty understanding jokes and sarcasm			
Difficulty with being creative or imaginative			
Other:			

Circle the feelings you have when there are problems with humor and imagination:

Frustrated   Confused   Annoyed   Embarrassed

Other: _____

Go through the following list of problem-solving skills together and check the ones you want to try:

☐   When people take things too literally or do not understand sarcasm, they can learn to say, "Did you mean that, or are you joking?" when they are not sure if they are understanding the meaning correctly.

☐ If your parent has difficulty with creative writing or imaginative projects, he or she can get someone else to help you with that type of homework. Someone else who might be good at helping is:

_____.

☐ If someone has difficulty understanding jokes, he or she can learn to say, "I didn't really get that joke. Can you please explain it?"

☐ If someone has difficulty understanding or telling jokes he or she can learn more about humor by reading joke books or watching comedy shows or sitcoms.

Chapter 12

Rules and Routines

NT children and teens often have ways they like to do things. When they get ready for school in the morning, they may follow a routine, such as first showering, then getting dressed, next eating breakfast and brushing their teeth, and lastly packing a backpack before going out to catch the bus. Their routines may be easy and comfortable for them. On the other hand, if there is some reason that the routine needs to change, they are able to be flexible with only some minor frustration. For instance, if all the hot water has been used up by their siblings, they would be able to eat breakfast and pack their backpacks before they shower while they wait for the water to heat up. They may feel most at ease with their regular teachers whom they have known for months, but if they have a substitute they can adjust. Sometimes they might even welcome the change of pace to get the chance to do things in a different way. They usually know the rules at school and home, but it may not be a big deal to them if the rules are not followed perfectly. That is, they may not view the rules as black or white but, instead, may be able to see the shades of gray. They may be able to see that something could be both partly right and partly wrong at the same time. NT children and teens may like it when they get to choose what to do when playing with friends, but they probably allow their friends to be in charge at times too.

What do you think it would be like for ASD children and teens when their routines are so important to them that they cannot be flexible when something different comes up? What if the thought of taking a shower after breakfast instead of before just seems impossible? What if dealing with the changes that a substitute teacher makes is overwhelming? What if they truly believe there is only one right way of doing things? Would this way of seeing things cause arguments? What if rules were so very important to them that they told adults when other children were not following them, and then the other children got angry and called them tattletales? What would the other kids think about them if they were bossy and demanding about doing things their way and did not let others take turns to be in charge?

People with ASDs often have fixed routines. Sometimes the routines make logical sense to others. For instance, it makes logical sense to others for people to shower first in the morning if they want to have more time for their hair to dry before they leave for the day. Other times the routines do not make logical sense to others but the person feels it has to be done that way regardless, such as eating the food on the plate in a particular order, all the while making sure none of the different food groups touch. There may be ASD adults who started following a routine that made logical sense when they were young (such as answering the phone in a certain way) but later, even though the routine no longer makes logical sense, they still continue following it in just the same way nevertheless. People with ASDs may be rigid in their thinking (seeing things as black or white, right or wrong), rather than flexible (seeing the shades of gray or that something can be both partly right and partly wrong). Because of this rigid thinking, children with ASDs may be seen as bossy when they are playing with others, and adults with ASDs may be seen as demanding or pushy at work or in their relationships.

My father is a master of routines! He has routines for showering, as I mentioned earlier in the book, and for getting ready in the morning. He even had a routine for how he mixed instant iced tea. First he turned on the faucet to start the cold water running so it would get cold. Then he measured out the instant tea and sugar with measuring spoons and put the precise amounts into the glass. Then he filled the glass part way up with water from the faucet. Then he added five ice cubes from the ice cube dispenser and stirred. Lastly he filled up the rest of the glass with water from the refrigerator door dispenser. We never knew why he filled part of the glass with water from the faucet and part of it with water from the refrigerator door, and so to the rest of us that routine did not make logical sense! Also, he is a "black or white" thinker when it comes to politics, and he truly believes that his position is the only smart and correct position and that other beliefs are both stupid and wrong. There are no grays or partial truths for my father when it comes to politics!

When I am counseling people with ASDs, I try to be careful about how I set up the first couple of therapy sessions. I know that the routine I set up is likely to become the only way for us to do therapy, even if another way of doing things would be helpful for us to try in the future. I also recommend that parents work with their ASD children when they are still young to set up routines that will be helpful in adulthood, such as taking a shower every day, doing their laundry, or setting their own alarm clocks, to help their children be more successful in the future.

Is your ASD parent also big on routines? If so, do you find that those routines work well or do they cause problems? Do you ever feel frustrated about your ASD parent being a "black or white" thinker without understanding shades of gray? When I was a child, I would get frustrated with my father's routines because they were so time consuming. I did not like waiting for him and did not understand why certain tasks that were quick for others took him so long to complete. Children tell me that it can lead to trouble when they want to do something a little differently than how their ASD parent wants it done. They may complain that their ASD parent is overly bossy or controlling.

Complete this worksheet with your family so you can all learn about each other and develop new skills to handle problems with rules and routines.

Rate how important routines are to you on a scale of 0 to 10:

0	1	2	3	4	5	6	7	8	9	10

Routines do   Routines
not matter   are very
much to me   important to
                                                              me

Have your ASD parent rate the importance of routines on a scale of 0 to 10:

0   1   2   3   4   5   6   7   8   9   10

Routines do   Routines
not matter   are very
much to me   important to
                                            me

If you have other family members, get their ratings.

Name of person: _____ Rating: _____

Name of person: _____ Rating: _____

Circle the feelings you have if there are problems in the family caused by too many routines:

Angry   Annoyed   Frustrated   Confused

Other: _____

Rate how black or white your thinking is on a scale of 0 to 10:

0   1   2   3   4   5   6   7   8   9   10

I am a   I can see
black or   shades of
white, all or   gray and
nothing thinker   partial truths

Have your ASD parent rate his or her thinking on the same scale from 0 to 10:

0   1   2   3   4   5   6   7   8   9   10

I am a   I can see
black or   shades of
white, all or   gray and
nothing thinker   partial truths

If you have other family members, get their ratings.

Name of person: _____ Rating: _____

Name of person: _____ Rating: _____

Go through the following list of problem-solving skills together and check the ones you want to try:

☐   If my parent has routines that are causing any family problems, a family meeting could be held to talk about those problems. We might be able to come up with new solutions that could make things go more smoothly.

☐   If my parent is too demanding, or is paying too much attention to rules, I can talk to my parent about my feelings using an "I-message" which goes like this: "When you are being too demanding or paying too much attention to rules, I feel

_____(the name of my feeling),

because _____.

I wish _____.

☐   If we have family problems over all or nothing thinking, we can try to find a middle path. We could try writing down different ways of seeing things, and the pros and cons of each of those ways of seeing things, and then see what we can come up with.

Chapter 13

Games and Sports

NT children and teens play many different games and sports. They may like it best when they win, but they know that they will lose at times and that when they do lose they should try to be "good sports." Being a good sport means congratulating the other team and not showing too much disappointment. They also know if they play on a team that they need to work hard not only to play their best, but also to get along with their team mates even if they do not like all of them. They know that they sometimes need to give up their chance to make a good play to give someone else a chance to make a good play. They get used to accepting feedback from team members and coaches about their weaknesses, and they know that even if the feedback hurts their feelings it is done to help them improve.

Being physically coordinated means that all the body parts work smoothly together to create movement. NT children and teens are different in how physically coordinated they are and how good they are at sports, but many of them are able to find sports at which they can do well or at least that they can enjoy. NT children and teens also usually know without thinking about it how to move their bodies in certain ways and how to balance.

ASD children and teens may find games and sports difficult. Since they may have difficulty getting along with others anyway, playing on a team can be especially hard. It can be hard for them to figure out how to play as a member of a team rather than just for themselves. If there is good-natured teasing going on they may misunderstand it and think that the others are being mean to them, and so react with anger. ASD children and teens may have a hard time accepting feedback about their weaknesses due to not understanding that others are trying to be helpful. They are known for having a hard time with losing games and not being able to hide their own personal disappointment.

ASD children and teens are also different in how physically coordinated they are. They are more likely than NTs to be clumsy because of the type of hardwiring they have (those neurological differences we talked about back in Chapter 3). This also means that when they are playing sports, they may end up with more than their share of negative feedback due to their clumsiness. ASD children and teens may have extra difficulty with knowing how their body is moving in space and with their sense of balance. Both of these issues can make it hard to be good at sports and other physical activities. Sometimes ASD children and teens work with physical therapists on ways to improve these coordination problems.

By the time ASD individuals have grown up, they have usually figured out if they are good at sports or not and are likely only to have continued with sports if it is an area of strength rather than weakness. Some people with ASDs find they do better in more individual sports such as swimming or martial arts rather than team sports such as soccer or basketball. Then they do not have to worry as much about getting along with the team members. Some ASD adults also have trouble seeing their children lose or getting negative feedback from a coach, and so they may have trouble being a good sport when their child or teen is involved in a game. Of course, there are NT parents who have some of these same issues! Additionally, some ASD parents find it hard to teach their children new sports, because they are not so good at sports themselves.

My father is physically well coordinated and tended to be successful in sports. When he was a child he liked to play baseball. However, since he does not like people very much he mostly played tennis when he got older and then he did not have to play on a team. He liked it best when he could play singles tennis (one player against one player) instead of doubles (two players against two). Then his focus could be on how well he played rather than on getting along with a tennis partner. When he did want to play doubles, other people sometimes refused to be his partner because they knew he might get mad at them and point out their mistakes too often. He also was not a good sport when he lost.

It is frequently mentioned to me that people with ASDs have trouble with their coordination. I remember one ASD teen telling me, "Balls and I just don't agree." Some have the worst time trying to catch and throw a ball! Others are slow to learn how to tie their shoes or to ride a bike. Even more often, it is brought up that people with ASDs are bad losers when they play sports or board games. Families affected by ASDs tell me that playing games at home can lead to arguments or meltdowns.

What is it like in your family? Does your ASD parent have any trouble with getting angry over losing a game or with being a bad sport? Has this problem ever caused you any embarrassment? When I was a child, I got to the point of not wanting to play games with my father because it was not enjoyable. He was very competitive and would usually win, so it stopped being fun for me. Children with ASD parents tell me that their parents are too intense about winning or losing. Also, they sometimes feel frustrated because they want to learn a new sport, but their ASD parent is not able to help them learn it because of his or her own coordination problems.

Complete this worksheet with your family so you can all learn about each other and develop new skills to handle problems with games and sports.

Rate how well you do at sports and how coordinated you are on a scale of 0 to 10:

0   1   2   3   4   5   6   7   8   9   10

One of   One of
my weak   my strong
points   points

Have your ASD parent rate how well he or she does at sports and how coordinated he or she is on a scale of 0 to 10:

0   1   2   3   4   5   6   7   8   9   10

One of   One of
my weak   my strong
points   points

If you have other family members, get their ratings.

Name of person: _____ Rating: _____

Name of person: _____ Rating: _____

Rate how well you handle losing on a scale of 0 to 10:

    0   1   2   3   4   5   6   7   8   9   10

It is hard   It is easy
for me to be   for me to be
a "good sport."   a "good sport."

Have your ASD parent rate him or herself on the same scale from 0 to 10:

    0   1   2   3   4   5   6   7   8   9   10

It is hard   It is easy
for me to be   for me to be
a "good sport."   a "good sport."

If you have other family members, get their ratings.

Name of person: _____ Rating: _____

Name of person: _____ Rating: _____

Circle the feelings you have if someone is your family has trouble being a good sport:

       Embarrassed   Sad   Angry   Worried

          Confused   Disappointed   Hurt

Other: _____

Go through the following list of problem-solving skills together and check the ones you want to try:

☐ When we play games as a family, we could choose cooperative games (games that require us to work together towards a goal) instead of competitive games (where one player or one team wins and the other loses).

☐ If someone is having trouble being a good sport, he or she can try hard to learn to congratulate the winner and accept losing gracefully, to make others feel comfortable playing games with him or her.

☐ When we want to exercise or play sports, we can find something that works for the whole family. Circle the activities we might enjoy trying: swimming, biking, walking, yoga, martial arts, weight lifting, others: _____.

☐ If I want to learn a sport at which my parent is not good, we can find someone else (a friend, a neighbor, a coach, or another family member) to help me learn it. A sport I would like to try is_____. A person who might be able to help me is _____.

Chapter 14

The Five Senses

The way we experience the world is through our senses. Our five senses are touch, taste, smell, hearing, and sight. We touch with our skin, we taste with our taste buds, we smell with our noses, we hear with our ears, and we see with our eyes. We know how difficult it can be for someone who is partly or completely blind, because those people are not able to experience the world with their sense of sight. We may know people who are partly or completely deaf and who are not able to experience the world with their sense of hearing. There are ways of helping people who are partly or completely blind or deaf. For instance, we know that people can wear glasses or use white canes or hearing aids. However, we may know less about what it is like for someone who experiences his or her senses in ways that are different, such as when the sensation is very weak or very strong.

What do you think it would be like if someone was patted on the back and the pat hurt so much that it made him or her cry, or if the tags on his or her clothes were so irritating that they always had to be cut out? ASD children and teens often experience the world through their senses in different or even painful ways. Sometimes their senses are overactive, and then they are likely to stay away from those types of feelings. Some examples of this are children and teens who do not like to be hugged because for them it might hurt instead of feel good, or those who cannot stand the taste or texture of certain foods and so might end up only being able to eat a few things. Some more examples are children who put their hands over their ears when they hear loud sounds such as a fire alarm drill, begin to gag in the school cafeteria because of all the smells, or do not like to go outside because the sunlight hurts their eyes. Sometimes their senses are underactive and they might either not notice those types of feelings or try to get more of those feelings. Some examples are children and teens who barely notice pain and therefore might not even know when they are sick and need to tell a parent, or those who want the feeling of something in their mouths and therefore put almost anything in their mouths! Children and teens with sensory differences might work with an occupational therapist to learn coping skills.

By the time people with ASDs are adults, some of them have got over their sensory differences. If not, they are usually well aware they have sensory issues and they are able to let others know what bothers them. Therefore, if your ASD parent has a sensory issue, you have probably heard him or her talk about it. You may have been told that sounds bother your ASD parent, or you may know he or she only likes to wear certain types of clothes because of the feel of the material against the skin. However, there are many NT people who have differences with their senses too so keep in mind that just having sensory differences does not mean that someone has an ASD; it is just more common for people with ASDs.

My father is one of the ASD adults who does not have any special sensory issues. I am one of the NT adults who is very sensitive about sounds, and I find it almost impossible to sleep if I am in a motel room with a noisy fan! I have known ASD adults who have to turn off the fluorescent light because of being bothered by the flickering. I usually keep my office decorated very simply and I put any clutter away into drawers or cabinets, so that those things do not overload my ASD clients. I also notice that my ASD clients get startled easily by the noises coming from nearby offices. If the fire alarm is going to sound in our waiting room as part of a drill, I like to let my ASD clients know ahead of time, in case they need to wait outside when it goes off.

Does your ASD parent, or anyone else in your family, have any of these types of sensory issues? Do these sensory issues cause any problems for you? Sometimes my own children complain they cannot do very much in the house when I go to bed early because the littlest sound will wake me up! Other children have told me that their ASD parents can only handle wearing certain types of clothes, such as sweat pants, so the kids end up feeling embarrassed about how their parents look. Others have complained that they cannot go out to eat in certain restaurants because their ASD parent cannot stand the smells.

Complete this worksheet with your family so you can all learn about each other and develop new skills to handle sensory problems.

Rate if you have any sensory differences on a scale of 0 to 10:

0	1	2	3	4	5	6	7	8	9	10

I do not
have
sensory
issues

I have
major
sensory
issues

If you do, circle the ones you have:

Touch   Taste   Smell   Hearing   Sight

Have your ASD parent rate his or her sensory differences on a scale of 0 to 10:

0	1	2	3	4	5	6	7	8	9	10

I do not
have
sensory
issues

I have
major
sensory
issues

If your ASD parent has sensory issues, have him or her circle which senses are affected:

Touch   Taste   Smell   Hearing   Sight

If you have other family members, get their ratings, and have them circle the sensory issues they have.

Name of person: _____ Rating: _____

Touch   Taste   Smell   Hearing   Sight

Name of person: _____ Rating: _____

Touch   Taste   Smell   Hearing   Sight

Circle the feelings you have when there are problems in the family with sensory issues:

Embarrassed   Annoyed   Frustrated

Confused   Worried

Other: _____

Go through the following list of skills together and check the ones that might help solve any sensory problems:

☐ We can keep the sound turned down low or wear headphones when watching TV or listening to music.

☐ We can play music during dinner so that other sounds such as the chewing noises will not bother anyone.

☐ If someone in the family does not like to be touched, we can ask before we touch him or her (such as asking before we give hugs or kisses).

☐ We can be careful not to use products that have strong smells around the house (such as cleaning products, air fresheners, scented candles, perfumes, aftershave, and so forth).

☐ We can be careful to use the kinds of lights in our home that do not bother anyone in the family.

☐ We can try to shop for and prepare food that everyone in the family enjoys.

Chapter 15

Telling Friends

Many children and teens who have an ASD in their family wonder whether to tell others about the ASD. When someone in a family is deaf or blind, we generally tell friends and neighbors. We do this so our deaf or blind family member can get the help he or she needs, and so that other people can understand our deaf or blind family member. When someone in the family is seriously ill, we usually tell our friends and neighbors, and then those friends and neighbors do things to help the family out such as bringing meals or giving the ill person a ride to the doctor's office.

An interesting thing happens when it comes to ASDs. Many people are nervous about talking about ASDs because of the stigma. A stigma means that something has a negative reputation. ASDs have a negative reputation in some people's eyes. For instance, it may be thought that all people with ASDs cannot talk or care for themselves. It may not be realized that a person with an ASD could also be a college professor, an engineer, a computer programmer, or a musician. It may not be known that there are many people with ASDs who are married, have children, have friends, and are successful at their jobs.

Because of this stigma, some people choose not to tell others about their ASD. They may only tell their family or a few close friends. Others who are diagnosed with ASDs are working to change the stigma of ASDs and like to let others know that they are "auties" (autistic) or "Aspies" (have Asperger's Syndrome). Still others do not think of themselves as having a disorder or a disability, as we talked about in Chapter 3, and think that how they think and see the world is just a normal human difference and not a problem at all. Those people may choose not to talk about the diagnosis for this reason, and they may be hurt if others talk about the ASD as a problem. Lastly, sometimes there is more than one person in the same family with an ASD, and they may not agree on whether they want the diagnosis talked about openly.

There are several important things for you to think about when it comes to telling other people about your parent's diagnosis. The first is how your parent wants you to handle this issue. You will be able to find out how your parent feels about it when you complete this chapter's worksheet. Another important thing to think about is whether you, your ASD parent, or anyone else in the family could get more support if it was openly discussed. If others know that someone in the family has an ASD they may be more sensitive and helpful about those differences. On the other hand, when others know they are not always more helpful because of the stigma we discussed earlier. A third important thing is how you feel about it. Some children and teens find that their friends ask them questions about their ASD parent or that they misunderstand their ASD parent. They would like to talk to their friends and get understanding and support, but they also do not want to hurt their parent's feelings.

If the diagnosis is shared with others, a decision needs to be made about what words are used to explain it. Some people are comfortable sharing the official diagnosis, but even if that is done, not everyone knows what "autism," "Asperger's Syndrome," "PDD.NOS," or "autism spectrum disorder" means. They may reply, "What's that?" or, as discussed earlier in this chapter, might have the wrong idea of what these terms mean. The term may have to be explained, maybe using some of the ideas we have talked about in this book. They might need to be told it means the person has trouble with social skills, or trouble "being in someone else's shoes," or dealing with change. When I was growing up, we did not know that my father had an ASD, so when we were in awkward situations due to his differences, we would explain the problem in other ways. We would say, "My father doesn't like to socialize." Sometimes my father would say to people himself, "I don't like small talk."

Complete this worksheet with your family so you can all learn about each other and develop new skills to handle problems about telling friends.

Circle the feelings you have about telling others about the ASD(s) in your family:

Nervous   Confused   Worried   Annoyed

Embarrassed   Sad   Happy

Other: _____

Here are some issues that children and teens think about when they have a parent with an ASD. Check the ones that are true for you, and share them with the rest of your family.

☐ Sometimes people ask me questions about why my ASD parent is acting differently.

☐ I feel embarrassed when my ASD parent acts differently.

☐ I sometimes feel I need to warn people that my ASD parent might act differently.

☐ I worry about what will happen if friends come over to my home or spend time with my family.

☐ I wish I could talk to my friends about these things so they would understand my family better.

☐ I wish I could meet some other people my age who have a parent with an ASD.

☐ I want to protect my ASD parent from others who might be negative.

Have your ASD parent check which sentence best describes him or her:

☐ I mostly keep my ASD diagnosis private. Here are the people who know:

_____

_____

_____

☐ I like telling people about my ASD diagnosis and teaching them about ASDs.

☐ I do not believe that I have a "disorder" so I don't like the whole idea of talking about ASDs as if they are a problem.

☐ I handle talking about it in this way: _____

_____

If there is anyone else in your family with an ASD, have them also check which sentences describe them best. If you have an ASD, check which sentence describes you best. If you have other family members that you would like to rate, add their details at the bottom of the page.

☐ I mostly keep my ASD diagnosis private. Here are the people who know:

_____

_____

_____

☐ I like telling people about my ASD diagnosis and teaching them about ASDs.

☐ I do not believe that I have a "disorder" so I don't like the whole idea of talking about ASDs as if they are a problem.

☐ I handle talking about it in this way: _____

_____

Chapter 16

Special Strengths and Contributions

NT children and teens have many different strengths and talents. One may be good at playing the piano, another may be a soccer player, while yet another may be the geography whiz of the class. These things are true about ASD children and teens too. One may be good at playing the organ, another may be a tennis player, while yet another may be the best in the class at math. However, we also know that people with ASDs are likely to share certain types of strengths that are linked to how their brains are wired. "Autistic" thinking has advantages. There are contributions that people with ASDs have made to the world that they would not have been able to make if they did not have this special way of thinking and of seeing the world.

For instance, many people with ASDs are very good logical thinkers. They might remind you of the character of Spock in the *Star Trek* series, because they can be so skilled at figuring things out. They also tend to be good at remembering details, facts, and figures. Do you know the character of Sherlock Holmes from Sir Arthur Conan Doyle's book *The Adventures of Sherlock Holmes*? Holmes was an expert at knowing unusual facts and as a detective he used his knowledge of these facts to solve crimes. Some people describe Sherlock Holmes as a good example of someone on the autism spectrum. Interestingly enough, some think that Sir Arthur Conan Doyle was himself on the autism spectrum.

Many people with ASDs have an excellent memory for things that happened in the past, such as events that happened many years ago that others have long forgotten. People with ASDs are also skilled at being able to see how things fit and work together. Children on the autism spectrum may demonstrate this skill by being good at puzzles. Adults on the autism spectrum may demonstrate this skill by being good at engineering or at computer programming.

People with ASDs tend to be honest, reliable, and fair, and they rarely lie. They are frequently law-abiding "good citizens" and may not like the idea of people breaking rules. They may make good police officers because of this quality! In general, people with ASDs have excellent focus if the topic interests them (especially if it is one of their special interests). There can also be good things about not worrying too much about others' feelings or about superficial things (such as how someone dresses). These good things include a willingness to say what you really think and not spending a lot of time or money on things that do not truly matter in life. People with ASDs are not as likely to want to spend time or money on their appearance because they look at the matter in a more logical manner than NTs, who get caught up in the social pressure to look a certain way.

There is one type of strength that is seen in just a very few people on the autism spectrum, but I will mention it because people are often curious about it. This is when someone is a "savant." Being a savant means that the person has one skill that is very highly developed while their other skills range from normal to below normal. In the film *Rain Man*, the actor Dustin Hoffman played the role of Raymond Babbitt, an autistic savant who had amazing math and memory skills while some of his other skills were below normal and he was not able to live on his own. There is also a man called Stephen Wiltshire from London, whose nickname is "The Living Camera." Stephen is able to see a city from a helicopter for 45 minutes and then draw an accurate and detailed picture of that city, including not only the layout of each and every road and building, but even the number of columns on each of the buildings. You can watch videos of his amazing ability on YouTube. However, it is reported that Stephen has autism and that he was not able to talk until he was five years old.

Now that people understand more about ASDs than they used to, they like to try to figure out which famous people throughout history might have had ASDs. There is a wonderful children's book about the scientist Albert Einstein (who lived from 1879 to 1955) called *Odd Boy Out: Young Albert Einstein*, which describes his childhood in a way that could be a description of a boy on the autism spectrum. Some other famous people who may have had ASDs are the US President Thomas Jefferson (1743–1826), the composer Wolfgang Amadeus Mozart (1756–1791), and the poet Emily Dickinson (1830–1886).

There are people on the autism spectrum who are very public about their autism and help to educate others about what it means to have autism. Temple Grandin is one of those people, and another is Jerry Newport. Temple is an author and professor, and she designs equipment for cattle. In 2010 the television station HBO made a movie about her called *Temple Grandin*. Jerry is an author with Asperger's Syndrome whose life was the basis for the 2005 movie *Mozart and the Whale*. Jerry is also a savant with the ability to perform extremely difficult math problems in his head.

Since my father always said what he thought, you knew where you stood with him. He did not try to pretend to be anyone different than who he really was, which is not something that all of us can say. He had amazing abilities in chess, almost to the point of being a "savant" in this area! One time he played 22 other players in a simultaneous blindfold chess exhibition. This means he played 22 other players at the same time, but he could not see the chessboards even though the other players could. There was someone called a teller helping him by telling him each of the other players' moves. He had to be able to "see" all 22 chessboards in his mind, including how each of the 22 positions changed with each move. Scientists who study human memory say that no other human memory accomplishment can beat the achievements of the best simultaneous blindfold chess champions!

What have you noticed about your ASD parent? Have you noticed any special skills or talents? Have there been times when you feel impressed with or proud of the accomplishments of your parent, or when you have thought about the special contributions your parent is making to your family or to your community? There may be things that you have learned or gained by having a parent with an ASD. Maybe your parent has taught you things or helped you understand what is really important in life. You may have developed a good understanding of all the different kinds of people we need to have in this world to make it the amazing place that it is!

Complete this worksheet with your family so you can all learn about each other and recognize each other's strengths and talents.

Read through this list of strengths and talents and have each family member put his or her initials next to the items that are true for him or her. Put your initials next to the statements that are true for you.

	You	Your ASD parent	Other family members
I am a very good logical thinker.	___	___	___ ___ ___
I am very good at remembering facts, figures, and details.	___	___	___ ___ ___
I have a very good long-term memory.	___	___	___ ___ ___
I am very good at understanding how things work.	___	___	___ ___ ___
I am very honest, reliable, and fair.	___	___	___ ___ ___
I am very good at following rules.	___	___	___ ___ ___
I am very good at saying exactly what I think.	___	___	___ ___ ___
I do not get caught up in the latest fashions and trends.	___	___	___ ___ ___
I can have very good focus in my areas of interest.	___	___	___ ___ ___

Do you know what a family coat of arms is? Coats of arms were symbols originally used on shields by feudal knights and lords to identify themselves in battle. Nowadays, a coat of arms can be used to celebrate the strengths or talents of each family member and identify the ways in which the family is special. Try to draw a family coat of arms that includes at least one strength of each member of your family in the space below.

Printed in Great Britain
by Amazon